The Complete Diabetic Diet After 50

Empowering Your Diet: A Comprehensive Guide to Nutritious Eating for Mature Adults with Diabetes

ANNE G. BARNEY

Table of Contents

Introduction

The Promise of Renewal: A Short Story on "The Complete Diabetic Diet After 50"

In the golden glow of a serene autumn afternoon, Eleanor, a spry 68-year-old with twinkling blue eyes, sat with her granddaughter under the old oak in her backyard. Over the years, the oak had witnessed many changes, much like Eleanor, who had recently been navigating the challenges of type 2 diabetes.

"Gran, why are you smiling like that?" asked Sarah, noticing Eleanor's content expression as she leafed through a well-worn book titled "The Complete Diabetic Diet After 50."

"This book, my dear," Eleanor began, her voice warm and steady, "is like a guide to a treasure map. It's helped me rediscover the joy of health, even after 50."

Curiosity piqued, Sarah leaned closer. "How so?"

"Well," Eleanor explained, "after your granddad passed, I let myself go. My blood sugar was all over the place, I felt tired all the time, and honestly, I was scared. Then, Dr. Linton recommended this book."

"The Complete Diabetic Diet After 50" was no ordinary diet guide; it was a beacon of hope for Eleanor. The book was meticulously organized into three main sections: breakfast, lunch, and dinner, each offering a variety of nutritious, easy-to-prepare recipes tailored for those managing diabetes in their golden years.

"What's so special about it?" Sarah inquired, intrigued by her grandmother's enthusiasm.

"It's not just a list of recipes; it's a lifestyle change," Eleanor replied. Each recipe was designed to stabilize blood sugar levels and provide all the necessary nutrients to stay healthy and energized. Eleanor had learned how to mix and match the right foods to keep her blood sugar balanced, something she struggled with after her diagnosis.

"See this?" Eleanor pointed at a bookmarked page. "This morning I made the 'Sunrise Berry Oatmeal'. It was delicious and kept my sugar level steady till lunch!"

Sarah watched as her grandmother turned the pages, showing her vibrant photos of meals and detailed nutritional information that included carb counts, protein amounts, and fats, all crucial for making informed dietary choices.

"But it's more than just food," Eleanor continued, a note of excitement in her voice. "The book talks about understanding our body's needs as we age. There's a whole section on how metabolism changes after 50 and what we can do to adapt."

The story took a more personal turn as Eleanor shared how the guide had helped her regain control of her health, allowing her more energy to play with her grandchildren, tend her garden, and even join a local walking group. "It gave me a part of my life back that I thought was over."

Sarah listened, her eyes reflecting a mix of pride and wonder. "Gran, I'm so glad you found this book. You seem so much happier."

"I am," Eleanor affirmed, her gaze affectionate. "And I want the same for anyone who thinks age or diabetes can stop them from living a full life. This book—it's a powerful tool. It teaches, guides, and encourages. It's about making the most of every meal, every day, and every moment after 50."

As the sun dipped lower, casting long shadows across the yard, Eleanor closed the book and smiled, her decision clear. "I think I'll gift this to Joan for her birthday. She's been struggling too, and if this can bring her even a fraction of the joy and health it's brought me, it'll be worth it."

Sarah nodded, her heart swelling with admiration. "You're amazing, Gran."

Together, they sat under the oak, talking about life, love, and recipes—a simple yet profound reminder of how the right guidance can lead to a life well-nourished and well-lived.

"The Complete Diabetic Guide After 50" isn't just a book; it's a companion in the journey toward health and happiness, proving that life after 50 can be vibrant and fulfilling.

Diabetes management post-50 presents unique challenges and necessitates adjustments to diet and lifestyle to maintain optimal health. As individuals age, the body's ability to manage blood sugar levels diminishes due to a natural decline in pancreatic function and insulin sensitivity. This stage of life often brings about a slower metabolism, making weight management more difficult and increasing the risk of type 2 diabetes. Thus, a tailored approach focusing on dietary adjustments becomes essential, as showcased in "The Complete Diabetic Diet After 50," which offers practical, easy-to-follow meal plans specifically designed for this age group.

The book emphasizes the importance of incorporating a balanced mix of nutrients in every meal to help stabilize blood sugar levels. Foods rich in fiber, such as vegetables, fruits, whole grains, and legumes, play a pivotal role in this diet. Fiber not only aids in digestion but also helps slow down the absorption of sugar, preventing spikes in blood glucose levels. Furthermore, these fiber-rich foods contribute to a feeling of fullness, which can help curb overeating and support weight management efforts, crucial for those managing diabetes.

Protein is another cornerstone of the dietary plan outlined in the book. Adequate protein intake is vital for muscle maintenance, especially important for older adults who are at risk of muscle loss. The guide provides creative ways to include lean protein sources like chicken, fish, tofu, and legumes in meals. These proteins do not significantly impact blood sugar levels and thus are ideal for a diabetic-friendly diet.

Understanding fats and their impact on health is another area the book covers comprehensively. It distinguishes between healthy fats, which can support heart health, and unhealthy fats, which should be limited. Recipes in the guide make liberal use of healthy fats found in nuts, seeds, avocados, and olive oil, which can help improve cholesterol levels and reduce inflammation, benefiting overall health and specifically cardiovascular health, which is a concern for those with diabetes.

Portion control is a critical aspect discussed, teaching readers how to measure and understand portion sizes, which can be particularly challenging when dietary restrictions are necessary. The guide offers practical tips on how to visually divide your plate to include appropriate portions of each food group, ensuring a balanced meal without the need to count calories obsessively.

Aside from dietary advice, the book also acknowledges the importance of regular physical activity in managing diabetes after 50. Regular exercise can improve insulin sensitivity, help in weight management, and boost overall energy levels. Whether it's walking, swimming, cycling, or any other form of moderate activity, incorporating movement into daily routines is strongly advocated for.

Finally, "The Complete Diabetic Diet After 50" does more than just provide meal plans and recipes; it serves as an educational tool that empowers readers to make informed choices about their health. It encourages routine monitoring of blood sugar levels, regular check-ups with healthcare providers, and staying informed about the condition. This holistic approach not only helps manage diabetes effectively but also enhances the overall quality of life, proving that a proactive approach to health can lead to a fulfilling and active lifestyle beyond the age of 50.

Maintaining a balanced diabetic diet is crucial, especially for individuals over 50, as it significantly impacts overall health and well-being. As the body ages, its metabolic rate slows down, and the ability to process sugar effectively diminishes. This makes older adults more susceptible to spikes in blood sugar levels, which can exacerbate the complications associated with diabetes, such as cardiovascular diseases, nerve damage, and kidney issues. A well-balanced diet, as outlined in "The Complete Diabetic Diet After 50," provides the necessary nutrients while managing carbohydrate intake to help stabilize blood sugar levels throughout the day.

This tailored diet focuses on incorporating a variety of foods that are low in glycemic index and rich in fiber. Foods like whole grains, leafy greens, and fresh fruits not only provide essential vitamins and minerals but also help in the slow release of glucose into the bloodstream, preventing sudden spikes. Protein sources such as lean meats, beans, and legumes play a pivotal role in this diet by providing energy and aiding muscle repair without affecting blood sugar levels significantly. Including healthy fats from sources like avocados, nuts, and olive oil is equally important as they contribute to heart health without impacting glucose levels.

Portion control is another fundamental aspect emphasized in the guide. Overeating, even healthy foods, can lead to weight gain and increased blood sugar. The guide provides practical tips on measuring portions and understanding the appropriate serving sizes for different food groups, which is especially helpful for those who may struggle with maintaining a healthy weight. This approach not only helps in managing diabetes but also aids in preventing obesity, which is a significant risk factor for developing type 2 diabetes.

Meal timing is also a critical component of a balanced diabetic diet. Eating at regular intervals throughout the day ensures that there is a steady supply of energy, which helps in maintaining stable blood sugar levels. It also prevents the temptation of snacking on unhealthy options or overeating during meals, which can disrupt blood sugar control. The guide encourages planning meals and snacks to align with the body's natural rhythms and medication schedules.

Furthermore, hydration plays an essential role in managing diabetes. Water helps in the regulation of blood sugar levels by enabling the kidneys to flush out excess glucose through urine. The guide highlights the importance of staying hydrated and provides alternatives like herbal teas and sugar-free beverages for those who might find consuming large amounts of water challenging.

Adjusting the diet to include seasonal and locally available foods can also enhance its nutritional value and ensure that individuals are getting the freshest and most beneficial options available. This not only supports local farmers but also adds variety to the diet, which is important for maintaining interest and enjoyment in meals. Seasonal foods often contain optimal levels of nutrients, which can provide additional health benefits.

In conclusion, adopting a balanced diabetic diet as described in "The Complete Diabetic Diet After 50" is vital for managing diabetes effectively in later life. It supports not only blood sugar control but also enhances overall health, providing a pathway to a vibrant and active lifestyle post-50. By focusing on balanced nutrition, portion control, meal timing, hydration, and the inclusion of seasonal foods, individuals can significantly improve their quality of life despite having diabetes.

Managing diabetes after the age of 50 can feel daunting due to metabolic changes, the need for more careful dietary considerations, and the common misconceptions about what it means to live with this condition in later life. "The Complete Diabetic Diet After 50" addresses these issues directly by providing tailored nutritional advice that respects the body's evolving needs. This guide emphasizes the importance of understanding how and why the body's response to food changes with age, offering practical strategies for adapting dietary habits to maintain healthy blood sugar levels.

The book's comprehensive approach helps readers identify foods that can naturally regulate blood glucose levels. Each recipe and meal plan is designed not only to satisfy taste buds but also to ensure that meals are balanced with the necessary nutrients that support an older adult's health. More importantly, these meals consider the glycemic index of foods, portion control, and how pairing certain foods can prevent blood sugar spikes, key concerns for anyone managing diabetes.

Beyond recipes, the guide delves into the psychological and emotional aspects of managing diabetes. It encourages readers to cultivate a positive relationship with food, which is crucial for long-term health management. The approach demystifies nutritional science, making it accessible and actionable. This empowers readers, making them feel more in control of their health, and reduces the anxiety that often accompanies a diabetes diagnosis.

The practical benefits of the book are clear. It helps in reducing dependency on medication by providing dietary choices that can complement medical treatments. This is particularly significant for those who are looking to manage their condition through lifestyle changes as much as possible. The book stresses the importance of consistency in eating habits, which can lead to significant improvements in overall health metrics such as weight, cholesterol levels, and insulin sensitivity.

For those who may feel isolated or overwhelmed by their dietary restrictions, this book also acts as a community bridge, sharing stories and testimonials from others who are navigating the same path. These narratives provide comfort and companionship, offering reassurance that one is not alone in this journey. They also serve to inspire and motivate readers to make and maintain the necessary changes for a healthier life.

Moreover, the book is an invaluable resource for family members and caregivers of older adults with diabetes. It educates them on the nutritional needs specific to this age group and the complexities of managing diabetes. This can improve the quality of support they provide, whether in meal preparation, grocery shopping, or emotional and moral support.

In conclusion, "The Complete Diabetic Diet After 50" is more than a dietary guide—it is a holistic tool for managing health that respects the challenges and embraces the possibilities of living with diabetes in one's golden years. By integrating nutritional science, practical advice, and empathetic support, it stands as an essential resource for anyone looking to lead a healthier and more balanced life despite their diabetic condition.

Chapter 1: The Basics of Diabetes Management

Key Nutrients and Their Roles

Understanding the key nutrients and their specific roles in managing diabetes is crucial, especially for those over 50. Carbohydrates often receive the most attention in diabetic diets because they have the most immediate effect on blood sugar levels. However, it's essential to focus on the type of carbohydrates consumed. Complex carbohydrates, like those found in whole grains, legumes, and vegetables, are integral to a diabetic diet as they are digested more slowly and cause a gradual rise in blood sugar, unlike their refined counterparts.

Proteins play a pivotal role as well, especially in the diet of an older adult with diabetes. As muscle mass tends to decrease with age, incorporating adequate protein can help maintain and build lean muscle, supporting metabolism and overall physical strength. Importantly, protein has minimal impact on blood sugar levels, making it a crucial component for stabilizing blood glucose throughout the day. Fish, lean meats, and plant-based sources like beans and lentils are excellent choices that offer both protein and other valuable nutrients without excessive calories or fats.

Fats are often misunderstood in the context of a healthy diet, but they are vitally important. For individuals managing diabetes, it's essential to focus on healthy fats that can help moderate blood sugar by slowing the absorption of carbohydrates. Sources like avocados, nuts, seeds, and olive oil not only provide healthy fats but also contribute to the feeling of fullness after meals, which can help control overall calorie intake.

Fiber is another cornerstone of a diabetic diet after 50, as it can help regulate blood sugar levels by slowing the digestion of carbohydrates and the absorption of sugar, helping to control blood glucose spikes. Soling fiber, found in foods like oats, peas, beans, apples, and carrots, can also help reduce cholesterol levels, a common concern for those with diabetes. Insoluble fiber, found in foods like whole grains and vegetables, aids digestion and prevents constipation, which can become more problematic as people age.

Vitamins and minerals also deserve attention in managing diabetes effectively. For instance, chromium plays a critical role in carbohydrate and fat metabolism and helps regulate blood sugar levels. It can be found in whole grains, nuts, and green beans. Similarly, magnesium, which is abundant in leafy greens, nuts, and whole grains, has been shown to improve insulin sensitivity, an essential factor in managing diabetes.

Water is an often-overlooked nutrient that plays a significant role in maintaining blood sugar levels. Adequate hydration helps in the efficient processing of glucose in the bloodstream and supports kidney function, which can be compromised in individuals with diabetes. Ensuring sufficient fluid intake is a simple yet effective way to support overall health and manage diabetes symptoms.

In conclusion, managing diabetes after 50 requires a balanced intake of carefully chosen nutrients that support metabolic health, enhance insulin sensitivity, and maintain muscle and digestive function. By focusing on a diet rich in complex carbohydrates, lean proteins, healthy fats, fiber, and essential vitamins and minerals, and ensuring adequate hydration, older adults can effectively manage their diabetes and enjoy a higher quality of life. Each of these nutrients plays a specific role in the overall management strategy, contributing to better health outcomes and reduced complications associated with diabetes.

Monitoring blood sugar levels is a fundamental aspect of managing diabetes, particularly for individuals over the age of 50. Regular checks allow for a clear understanding of how different foods, activities, and other factors such as stress affect glucose levels. This knowledge is crucial in preventing the highs and lows that can accompany poorly managed diabetes. By tracking these levels, individuals can make informed decisions about their diet and lifestyle, adjusting as necessary to maintain a stable condition.

The process involves using a blood glucose meter, a device that can provide a blood sugar reading from a small drop of blood. This test is typically performed multiple times a day, depending on the individual's treatment plan. For those following "The Complete Diabetic Diet After 50," the consistency of testing becomes an integral part of the routine, helping to gauge the effectiveness of the dietary strategies outlined in the book. The feedback from regular monitoring can lead to more personalized adjustments in the diet, ensuring meals are optimally balanced for sugar control.

Moreover, frequent monitoring can help detect patterns in blood sugar fluctuations. For instance, if readings consistently show elevated levels after consuming certain types of foods, individuals can consult the guide to find suitable alternatives that have a more balanced impact on their blood sugar. Conversely, if levels drop too low, it may be an indication that meals are too sparse in carbohydrates or the timing of meals needs adjustment, both of which are addressed in the diet guide.

Long-term adherence to a monitoring regimen not only helps in managing daily blood sugar levels but also aids in reducing the risk of developing complications associated with diabetes, such as neuropathy, retinopathy, and cardiovascular disease. These conditions are particularly concerning for older adults, as they can significantly impair quality of life. Thus, regular blood sugar monitoring is essential for maintaining overall health and preventing the long-term consequences of diabetes.

The feedback loop created by consistent blood sugar testing and dietary adjustments forms the cornerstone of effective diabetes management. It empowers individuals by providing tangible evidence of how their body responds to their diet and lifestyle choices. This empowerment is a central theme in "The Complete Diabetic Diet After 50," which emphasizes taking proactive steps to manage one's health through informed decision-making.

In addition to self-monitoring, regular consultations with healthcare providers are recommended. These professionals can offer insights into the data collected from blood sugar tests, suggest modifications to the diet, and provide medical interventions if necessary. Such partnerships ensure that the management plan remains effective and responsive to the changing health needs of the individual as they age.

Ultimately, monitoring blood sugar levels is about more than just keeping tabs on daily figures; it's about creating a lifestyle that supports sustained health and wellness. For those navigating diabetes after 50, integrating this practice with the guidance provided in "The Complete Diabetic Diet After 50" offers a comprehensive approach to managing their condition, enabling them to lead a full and active life despite the challenges posed by diabetes.

Adjusting Your Diet to Manage Diabetes

Adjusting your diet to effectively manage diabetes, especially after the age of 50, requires a deep understanding of how foods affect blood glucose levels. It is essential to focus on a balanced intake of nutrients that can help stabilize these levels while providing sufficient energy and maintaining overall health. Carbohydrates have the most direct impact on blood sugar, and learning to select the right type and amount of carbohydrates is foundational. Complex carbohydrates found in whole grains, legumes, and vegetables are preferable because they are digested more slowly, thus providing a gradual release of sugar into the bloodstream.

Protein is another crucial component of a diabetic diet. It helps to maintain muscle mass, which can be a concern for older adults. Moreover, protein does not raise blood glucose levels like carbohydrates do; however, it needs to be consumed in moderation to prevent overburdening the kidneys, which can be a concern in older individuals, particularly those with diabetes complications. Including lean protein sources like chicken, fish, tofu, and legumes in your diet is advisable. These provide essential nutrients without the added fats that can contribute to cardiovascular problems, another common concern for diabetic individuals.

Fats should not be overlooked, as they play a significant role in heart health and satiety. Opting for healthy fats such as avocados, nuts, seeds, and olive oil can help improve cholesterol levels and stabilize heart functions. It's important to limit the intake of saturated and trans fats, which can exacerbate heart conditions and increase the risk of diabetes-related complications. Balancing the types of fat in your diet can also help manage your weight, a key aspect of diabetes control.

Regular meal timing is another critical element in managing diabetes. Eating at regular intervals helps prevent significant fluctuations in blood sugar levels, which can be particularly hazardous for older adults. It is recommended to plan meals and snacks around the same time each day and to not skip meals. Portion control is equally important, as overeating can lead to weight gain and increased blood sugar levels, complicating diabetes management.

Hydration plays an often underestimated role in managing diabetes. Adequate water intake helps in the regulation of blood sugar levels and prevents dehydration, a risk when blood glucose levels are high. Limiting beverages that contain high amounts of sugars and artificial sweeteners is crucial; instead, water, unsweetened tea, and other non-caloric drinks are preferred choices.

Physical activity, in tandem with dietary adjustments, forms a comprehensive approach to managing diabetes. Exercise helps in maintaining a healthy weight, reduces blood sugar levels, and increases insulin sensitivity, meaning your body can better utilize the sugar in your bloodstream. For those over 50, it's essential to choose activities that are feasible and enjoyable, which encourages regularity and consistency.

Lastly, monitoring blood glucose levels is imperative to understand how different foods and activities affect your body. Regular checking can help you adjust your diet and lifestyle to better manage your diabetes. This continuous feedback loop allows for more precise control over your condition, reducing the risk of complications and improving overall quality of life. The Complete Diabetic Diet After 50 serves as a vital tool in guiding these adjustments, ensuring that dietary changes are not only effective in managing diabetes but also sustainable and aligned with the nutritional needs of aging adults.

Chapter 2: Breakfast Foods for Diabetics

Greek Yogurt with Berries and Flaxseeds

Ingredients:

- 1 cup plain Greek yogurt (non-fat or low-fat)
- 1/2 cup mixed berries (blueberries, strawberries, raspberries)
- 1 tablespoon ground flaxseeds
- Optional: A drizzle of honey or a sprinkle of cinnamon for added flavor

Instructions:

1. In a serving bowl, add one cup of Greek yogurt.
2. Top the yogurt with half a cup of freshly washed mixed berries.
3. Sprinkle one tablespoon of ground flaxseeds over the berries.
4. If desired, drizzle a small amount of honey or sprinkle cinnamon on top for extra flavor.
5. Gently mix all the ingredients together before serving if preferred, or serve layered.

Cooking Time: None required.

Serving Size: 1 serving

Nutritional Information:

- Calories: 190
- Total Fat: 4g
- Saturated Fat: 1g
- Cholesterol: 10mg
- Sodium: 65mg
- Total Carbohydrates: 19g
- Dietary Fiber: 3g
- Sugars: 15g (natural sugars from berries and yogurt, optional honey adds extra)
- Protein: 20g

Ingredients:

- 1 cup steel-cut oats
- 4 cups water
- 1 pinch salt
- 2 medium apples, peeled and sliced
- 1 tsp ground cinnamon
- 2 tbsp chopped walnuts (optional)
- 1 tbsp flaxseed meal (optional)
- Sugar substitute to taste

Instructions:

1. In a medium saucepan, bring the water to a boil. Add a pinch of salt and steel-cut oats. Reduce the heat to a simmer.
2. Cover and cook for 20 minutes, stirring occasionally. If you prefer a softer texture, cook for an additional 10 minutes.
3. While the oats are cooking, prepare the apples. In a separate pan, sauté the apple slices with cinnamon until they are soft and release their natural sugars, about 5-7 minutes.
4. Once the oats are cooked, remove from heat. Stir in the sautéed apple slices, walnuts, flaxseed meal, and sugar substitute.
5. Serve warm.

Nutritional Information (per serving):

- Calories: 250

- Total Fat: 5g
- Saturated Fat: 0.5g
- Cholesterol: 0mg
- Sodium: 70mg
- Total Carbohydrates: 45g
- Dietary Fiber: 8g
- Sugars: 10g (includes 0g added sugars)
- Protein: 7g

Serving Size: 1 cup

Cooking Time: 30 minutes

Whole Grain Avocado Toast

Ingredients:

- 2 slices whole grain bread
- 1 ripe avocado
- Pinch of salt
- Pinch of black pepper
- Optional toppings: sliced tomatoes, radishes, or a sprinkle of crushed red pepper flakes

Instructions:

1. Toast the whole grain bread slices to your desired level of crispness in a toaster or on a skillet over medium heat.
2. While the bread is toasting, cut the avocado in half, remove the pit, and scoop the flesh into a bowl.
3. Mash the avocado with a fork until it reaches a creamy, yet slightly chunky consistency. Season with salt and pepper to taste.
4. Spread the mashed avocado evenly over the toasted bread slices.
5. Add any optional toppings you like, such as sliced tomatoes, radishes, or a sprinkle of red pepper flakes for a bit of spice.

Nutritional Information:

- Calories: 290
- Total Fat: 15 g
- Saturated Fat: 2 g
- Cholesterol: 0 mg

- Sodium: 320 mg
- Total Carbohydrates: 34 g
- Dietary Fiber: 10 g
- Sugars: 4 g
- Protein: 9 g

Serving Size: 1 serving consists of 2 avocado toast slices.

Cooking Time: Approximately 5 minutes.

Ingredients:

- 2 large eggs
- 1 cup fresh spinach, washed and chopped
- 1 tablespoon olive oil
- Salt and pepper to taste
- Optional: 1 tablespoon grated Parmesan cheese

Instructions:

1. Heat olive oil in a non-stick skillet over medium heat.
2. Add the chopped spinach and sauté for 2-3 minutes until wilted.
3. In a bowl, beat the eggs with salt and pepper. Pour over the spinach in the skillet.
4. Stir gently to combine. Allow the eggs to set at the edges, then gently stir with a spatula to create soft curds.
5. Continue cooking until the eggs are fully cooked but still moist, about 3-4 minutes.
6. Sprinkle with Parmesan cheese if using, and serve immediately.

Nutritional Information:

- Calories: 230
- Total Fat: 18g
- Saturated Fat: 4g
- Cholesterol: 370mg

- Sodium: 220mg
- Total Carbohydrates: 2g
- Dietary Fiber: 1g
- Sugars: 1g
- Protein: 14g

Serving Size: 1 serving

Cooking Time: 10 minutes

Almond Butter and Banana Smoothie

Ingredients:

- 1 medium ripe banana
- 2 tablespoons almond butter (unsweetened)
- 1 cup unsweetened almond milk
- 1/2 cup Greek yogurt (low-fat)
- 1 tablespoon flaxseeds
- 1/2 teaspoon vanilla extract
- Ice cubes (optional)

Instructions:

1. Place the banana, almond butter, almond milk, Greek yogurt, flaxseeds, and vanilla extract into a blender.
2. Add a handful of ice cubes if you prefer a colder smoothie.
3. Blend on high speed until smooth and creamy.
4. Pour into a glass and serve immediately.

Nutritional Information:

- Calories: 280
- Protein: 10g
- Carbohydrates: 24g
- Fiber: 5g
- Sugar: 12g (natural sugars from banana)
- Fat: 16g
- Sodium: 95mg

Serving Size: 1 smoothie (approximately 1.5 cups)

Cooking Time: 5 minutes

Cottage Cheese with Pineapple
Chunks

Ingredients:

- 1 cup low-fat cottage cheese
- 1/2 cup fresh pineapple chunks
- 1 tablespoon chia seeds (optional)

Instructions:

1. In a serving bowl, place the low-fat cottage cheese.

2. Top with fresh pineapple chunks. Avoid canned pineapple as it may contain added sugars.

3. Sprinkle chia seeds on top for an extra boost of fiber and omega-3 fatty acids (optional).

4. Mix gently and serve immediately for the best taste and texture.

Nutritional Information (per serving):

- Calorics: 180
- Total Fat: 2g
- Saturated Fat: 1g
- Cholesterol: 10mg
- Sodium: 500mg
- Total Carbohydrates: 20g
- Dietary Fiber: 2g
- Sugars: 16g (natural sugars from pineapple)

- Protein: 20g

Serving Size: 1 bowl

Cooking Time: None (preparation time approximately 5 minutes)

Ingredients:

- 1 cup quinoa, rinsed
- 2 cups water
- 1 cup unsweetened almond milk
- 1 teaspoon cinnamon
- 1 tablespoon honey or a sweetener suitable for diabetics (such as stevia)
- Fresh berries or sliced fruit for topping
- Chopped nuts (optional)

Instructions:

1. In a medium saucepan, combine quinoa and water. Bring to a boil over high heat.
2. Reduce heat to low, cover, and simmer for 15 minutes, or until the water is absorbed and quinoa is tender.
3. Stir in almond milk, cinnamon, and honey or sweetener. Simmer for an additional 5 minutes, stirring occasionally.
4. Remove from heat and let sit for a couple of minutes to thicken.
5. Serve warm, topped with fresh berries or fruit and optional nuts for added texture and protein.

Nutritional Information (per serving):

- Calories: 210

- Protein: 6g
- Fat: 4g
- Carbohydrates: 38g
- Fiber: 5g
- Sugars: 7g (includes natural sugars from the fruit and any added sweeteners)

Serving Size:

- Makes 4 servings

Cooking Time:

- Prep time: 5 minutes
- Cook time: 20 minutes

Ingredients:

- 3 large eggs
- 1/4 cup diced turkey breast (cooked)
- 1/4 cup chopped bell peppers (mixed colors)
- 1/4 cup chopped onions
- 1/4 cup chopped spinach
- 2 tbsp shredded low-fat cheese
- 1 tbsp olive oil
- Salt and pepper to taste

Instructions:

1. Heat olive oil in a non-stick skillet over medium heat.

2. Add the onions and bell peppers, sautéing until they are soft, about 3-4 minutes.

3. Add the chopped spinach and cooked turkey breast to the skillet. Stir well and cook for an additional 2 minutes.

4. Beat the eggs in a bowl, season with salt and pepper, and pour over the sautéed vegetables and turkey in the skillet.

5. Cook over medium heat until the edges start to lift from the skillet. Sprinkle the shredded cheese over the omelette.

6. Carefully fold the omelette in half and continue cooking for another minute or until the cheese is melted and the eggs are cooked through.

7. Serve hot.

Nutritional Information (per serving):

- Calories: 320
- Total Fat: 20g
- Saturated Fat: 5g
- Cholesterol: 370mg
- Sodium: 330mg
- Total Carbohydrates: 6g
- Dietary Fiber: 1g
- Sugars: 3g
- Protein: 28g

Serving Size: 1 omelette

Cooking Time: 10-15 minutes

Ricotta Cheese and Pear Spread on
Whole Grain Toast

Ingredients:

- 2 slices of whole grain bread
- 1/2 cup ricotta cheese
- 1 ripe pear, thinly sliced
- 1/4 teaspoon ground cinnamon
- 1 tablespoon honey (optional)

Instructions:

1. Toast the whole grain bread slices to your preferred level of crispness.
2. In a small bowl, mix the ricotta cheese with cinnamon and honey (if using) until well combined.
3. Spread the ricotta mixture evenly over the toasted bread slices.
4. Top each slice with thin pear slices, arranging them in an even layer.
5. Serve immediately for best texture and flavor.

Nutritional Information (per serving):

- Calories: 270
- Protein: 12g
- Carbohydrates: 39g
- Fat: 8g

- Fiber: 6g
- Sugar: 18g (includes 6g added sugars if using honey)

Serving Size: 1 prepared toast

Cooking Time: 5 minutes

Ingredients:

- 1/4 cup chia seeds
- 1 cup unsweetened almond milk
- 1 tablespoon maple syrup (optional, for a touch of sweetness)
- 1/2 teaspoon vanilla extract
- 1/4 cup mixed nuts (almonds, walnuts, and pecans), chopped
- Fresh berries for topping (optional)

Instructions:

1. In a mixing bowl, combine the chia seeds, almond milk, maple syrup, and vanilla extract. Stir well to combine.
2. Cover the bowl and refrigerate for at least 2 hours, or overnight, allowing the chia seeds to absorb the liquid and form a pudding-like consistency.
3. Once the pudding is set, give it a good stir to break up any clumps.
4. Top with chopped mixed nuts and fresh berries if desired.

Nutritional Information:

- Calories: 295
- Total Fat: 18g
- Saturated Fat: 2g
- Cholesterol: 0mg
- Sodium: 65mg

- Total Carbohydrates: 27g

- Dietary Fiber: 10g

- Sugars: 10g (natural sugars from the ingredients)

- Protein: 8g

Serving Size: 1 serving

Cooking Time: 2 hours (mostly inactive time for soaking)

Chapter 3: Lunch Foods for Diabetics

Grilled Chicken Salad with Mixed Greens

Ingredients:

- 2 boneless, skinless chicken breasts
- 1 tablespoon olive oil
- 1 teaspoon dried oregano
- Salt and pepper to taste
- 4 cups mixed greens (lettuce, spinach, arugula)
- 1/2 cup cherry tomatoes, halved
- 1/4 cup sliced cucumbers
- 1/4 cup red onion, thinly sliced
- 1/4 cup crumbled feta cheese
- 2 tablespoons balsamic vinegar

Instructions:

1. Preheat grill to medium-high heat. Rub chicken breasts with olive oil, oregano, salt, and pepper.
2. Grill chicken for 6-7 minutes on each side or until fully cooked (internal temperature should reach 165°F). Remove from grill and let rest for a few minutes before slicing.

3. In a large bowl, combine mixed greens, cherry tomatoes, cucumbers, and red onion.

4. Add sliced grilled chicken to the salad.

5. Sprinkle feta cheese over the top.

6. Drizzle with balsamic vinegar and toss lightly to combine.

7. Serve immediately.

Nutritional Information (per serving):

- Calories: 290
- Fat: 15g
- Carbohydrates: 10g
- Fiber: 2g
- Protein: 30g

Serving Size: 1 serving

Cooking Time: 15 minutes (Prep Time: 5 minutes, Cook Time: 10 minutes)

Ingredients:

- 1 cup dried lentils, rinsed and drained
- 1/2 cup pearl barley
- 1 large carrot, diced
- 1 medium onion, chopped
- 2 cloves garlic, minced
- 1 stalk celery, diced
- 1 teaspoon dried thyme
- 1/2 teaspoon black pepper
- 1 bay leaf
- 4 cups low-sodium vegetable broth
- 2 cups water
- 1 tablespoon olive oil
- Salt to taste

Instructions:

1. Heat the olive oil in a large pot over medium heat. Add the onion, garlic, carrot, and celery. Sauté until the vegetables are tender, about 5-7 minutes.

2. Add the lentils, barley, thyme, black pepper, bay leaf, vegetable broth, and water to the pot. Stir to combine.

3. Bring the mixture to a boil, then reduce the heat to low and cover the pot. Let it simmer for about 45 minutes, or until the lentils and barley are fully cooked and tender.

4. Remove the bay leaf and season the soup with salt to taste.

5. If desired, use an immersion blender to partially blend the soup for a thicker consistency. Alternatively, leave it as is for a more textured soup.

Nutritional Information (per serving):

- Calories: 210
- Protein: 9g
- Fat: 3g
- Carbohydrates: 38g
- Fiber: 9g
- Sodium: 120mg

Serving Size: 1 cup

Cooking Time: Approximately 50 minutes

Turkey Wrap with Whole Wheat
Tortilla

Ingredients:

- 1 whole wheat tortilla (8-inch)
- 3 ounces of thinly sliced turkey breast
- 1/4 cup fresh spinach leaves
- 2 slices of ripe tomato
- 1 tablespoon low-fat mayonnaise
- 1 tablespoon mustard
- 1/4 avocado, thinly sliced
- 1/4 red onion, thinly sliced
- Salt and pepper to taste

Instructions:

1. Lay the whole wheat tortilla flat on a clean surface.

2. Spread the low-fat mayonnaise and mustard evenly over the tortilla.

3. Arrange the turkey slices in the center of the tortilla.

4. Add the spinach leaves, tomato slices, avocado, and red onion over the turkey.

5. Season with salt and pepper.

6. Carefully roll the tortilla tightly around the fillings, ensuring the ingredients are well enclosed.

7. Slice the wrap in half diagonally and serve immediately.

Nutritional Information:

- Calories: 320
- Total Fat: 9g
- Saturated Fat: 2g
- Cholesterol: 35mg
- Sodium: 480mg
- Total Carbohydrates: 35g
- Dietary Fiber: 5g
- Sugars: 3g
- Protein: 20g

Serving Size: 1 wrap

Cooking Time: 10 minutes

Ingredients:

- 1 cup quinoa, uncooked
- 2 cups water
- 1 can (15 ounces) black beans, rinsed and drained
- 1 medium red bell pepper, finely chopped
- 1/4 cup fresh cilantro, chopped
- 1/4 cup lime juice
- 2 tablespoons olive oil
- 1 teaspoon ground cumin
- 1/2 teaspoon salt (optional, based on dietary needs)
- 1/4 teaspoon black pepper
- 1/2 cup red onion, finely chopped
- 1 avocado, diced (optional)

Instructions:

1. Rinse quinoa under cold running water until water runs clear. Combine quinoa and water in a medium saucepan. Bring to a boil over high heat, then reduce heat to low, cover, and simmer for about 15 minutes or until all water is absorbed.
2. Remove from heat and let stand covered for 5 minutes. Fluff with a fork and allow to cool slightly.
3. In a large bowl, combine cooled quinoa, black beans, red bell pepper, red onion, and cilantro.

4. In a small bowl, whisk together lime juice, olive oil, cumin, salt, and black pepper. Pour over the quinoa mixture and toss to coat evenly.

5. If using, gently fold in diced avocado just before serving.

6. Serve chilled or at room temperature.

Nutritional Information (per serving):

- Calories: 200
- Protein: 8g
- Fat: 7g (with avocado increases to 10g)
- Carbohydrates: 30g
- Fiber: 8g
- Sodium: 300mg (varies with salt usage)

Serving Size: 1 cup

Cooking Time: 20 minutes prep, 15 minutes cooking, 35 minutes total.

Ingredients:

- 4 salmon fillets (6 ounces each)
- 2 tablespoons olive oil
- 1 teaspoon garlic powder
- Salt and pepper to taste
- 4 cups of broccoli florets
- 1 tablespoon lemon juice
- Optional: Fresh dill or parsley for garnish

Instructions:

1. Preheat your grill to medium-high heat. While the grill is heating, brush both sides of the salmon fillets with olive oil and sprinkle with garlic powder, salt, and pepper.
2. Place the salmon on the grill, skin-side down, and cover. Cook for about 6-8 minutes on each side, or until the salmon is opaque and flakes easily with a fork.
3. Meanwhile, steam the broccoli. Bring about an inch of water to a boil in a pot with a steaming basket. Add the broccoli, cover, and steam for about 5-7 minutes until tender but still crisp.
4. Once cooked, sprinkle the broccoli with lemon juice, and season with salt and pepper to taste.
5. Serve the grilled salmon with the steamed broccoli on the side. Garnish with fresh dill or parsley if desired.

Nutritional Information (per serving):

- Calories: 350
- Total Fat: 20g
- Saturated Fat: 3g
- Cholesterol: 70mg
- Sodium: 200mg
- Total Carbohydrates: 8g
- Dietary Fiber: 3g
- Sugars: 2g
- Protein: 34g

Serving Size: 1 salmon fillet with 1 cup of steamed broccoli

Cooking Time: 15-16 minutes

Ingredients:

- 1 lb lean beef, thinly sliced (preferably flank steak or sirloin)
- 2 cups broccoli florets
- 1 red bell pepper, sliced into thin strips
- 1 medium carrot, thinly sliced
- 2 cloves garlic, minced
- 2 teaspoons grated fresh ginger
- 2 tablespoons low-sodium soy sauce
- 1 tablespoon sesame oil
- 1 tablespoon olive oil
- 2 teaspoons cornstarch
- 1/4 cup water
- Salt and pepper to taste
- Fresh scallions and sesame seeds for garnish (optional)

Instructions:

1. In a small bowl, mix the cornstarch with water until smooth. Set aside.

2. Heat the olive oil in a large skillet or wok over medium-high heat. Add the beef in a single layer and stir-fry for about 2-3 minutes or until browned and nearly cooked through. Remove the beef from the skillet and set aside.

3. In the same skillet, add the sesame oil. When hot, add the broccoli, bell pepper, and carrot. Stir-fry for about 4-5 minutes until the vegetables are just tender but still crisp.

4. Add the garlic and ginger to the skillet and cook for an additional minute until fragrant.

5. Return the beef to the skillet. Add the soy sauce and the cornstarch mixture. Stir well to combine all ingredients and coat everything evenly. Continue to cook for another 2-3 minutes until the sauce has thickened and everything is heated through.

6. Season with salt and pepper to taste. Garnish with scallions and sesame seeds if using.

Nutritional Information:

- Calories: 280 per serving
- Carbohydrates: 12g
- Protein: 25g
- Fat: 16g
- Sodium: 330mg
- Fiber: 3g

Serving Size: 1 cup

Cooking Time: 15 minutes

Ingredients:

- 14 oz firm tofu, drained and cubed
- 1 tbsp olive oil
- 1 large onion, chopped
- 2 cloves garlic, minced
- 1 tbsp fresh ginger, grated
- 1 red bell pepper, diced
- 1 zucchini, sliced
- 1 yellow squash, sliced
- 2 tbsp curry powder
- 1 tsp turmeric
- 1/2 tsp cumin
- 1 can (14 oz) coconut milk
- 1 can (14 oz) diced tomatoes
- Salt and pepper, to taste
- 1/4 cup fresh cilious or basil for garnish

Instructions:

1. Heat the olive oil in a large skillet over medium heat. Add the onion, garlic, and ginger, sautéing until the onion becomes translucent.

2. Stir in the bell pepper, zucchini, and yellow squash, cooking for about 5 minutes or until they start to soften.

3. Sprinkle in the curry powder, turmeric, and cumin, stirring well to coat the vegetables.

4. Pour in the coconut milk and diced tomatoes, bringing the mixture to a gentle simmer. Let it cook for 10 minutes.

5. Gently fold in the tofu cubes, being careful not to break them. Season with salt and pepper.

6. Continue to simmer for an additional 10 minutes to allow flavors to meld.

7. Serve hot, garnished with fresh cilious or basil.

Nutritional Information:

- Calories: 250
- Total Fat: 18g
- Saturated Fat: 10g
- Cholesterol: 0mg
- Sodium: 200mg
- Total Carbohydrate: 15g
- Dietary Fiber: 4g
- Sugars: 6g
- Protein: 12g

Serving Size: 1 cup

Cooking Time: 30 minutes

Ingredients:

- 4 large Portobello mushrooms, stems removed
- 2 cups fresh spinach, chopped
- 1/2 cup feta cheese, crumbled
- 1/4 cup onions, finely chopped
- 2 cloves garlic, minced
- 1 tablespoon olive oil
- 1/2 teaspoon salt
- 1/4 teaspoon black pepper
- 1/4 cup low-sodium vegetable broth
- 2 tablespoons balsamic vinegar
- 1/4 teaspoon dried oregano

Instructions:

1. Preheat the oven to 375°F (190°C).
2. In a large skillet over medium heat, heat the olive oil. Add onions and garlic, sautéing until onions are translucent, about 3-4 minutes.
3. Add spinach to the skillet and cook until wilted, approximately 2-3 minutes. Remove from heat.
4. In a bowl, combine the sautéed spinach mixture, feta cheese, salt, pepper, and oregano.

5. Arrange the Portobello mushrooms on a baking sheet. Spoon the spinach and feta mixture evenly into the mushroom caps.

6. Pour vegetable broth and balsamic vinegar over the stuffed mushrooms.

7. Bake in the preheated oven until the mushrooms are tender, about 20-25 minutes.

Nutritional Information (per serving):

- Calories: 180
- Protein: 8 g
- Carbohydrates: 12 g
- Fat: 12 g
- Fiber: 3 g
- Sodium: 450 mg

Serving Size: 1 stuffed mushroom

Cooking Time: 25 minutes

Ingredients:

- 1 head of cauliflower, grated into rice-sized pieces
- 1 lb of large shrimp, peeled and deveined
- 2 tablespoons of olive oil
- 1 clove garlic, minced
- 1 lemon, juiced and zested
- 1/4 teaspoon of red pepper flakes (optional)
- Salt and pepper, to taste
- Fresh parsley, chopped (for garnish)

Instructions:

1. **Preparation of Cauliflower Rice:**

   - Rinse the cauliflower head and pat dry.

   - Remove the stems and use a box grater or food processor to grate the cauliflower into rice-sized pieces.

   - Heat a large skillet over medium heat and add one tablespoon of olive oil.

   - Add the grated cauliflower to the skillet, stirring occasionally. Cook for about 5-7 minutes until the cauliflower is tender but not mushy. Season with salt and pepper to taste.

2. **Grilling the Shrimp:**

- In a bowl, mix the shrimp with the remaining olive oil, minced garlic, lemon juice, zest, and red pepper flakes. Season with salt and pepper.
    - Preheat the grill to medium-high heat.
    - Thread the shrimp onto skewers and place them on the grill.
    - Grill the shrimp for 2-3 minutes per side or until they are pink and opaque.

3. **Combining and Serving:**
    - Serve the grilled shrimp over the bed of cauliflower rice.
    - Garnish with fresh parsley and extra lemon wedges on the side.

Nutritional Information:

- Calories: 250 per serving
- Protein: 24 g
- Carbohydrates: 8 g
- Fat: 14 g
- Fiber: 3 g
- Sugar: 2 g

Serving Size:

- This recipe serves 4 people.

Cooking Time:

- Total time: 30 minutes (Prep time: 15 minutes, Cook time: 15 minutes)

Ingredients:

- 1 can (15 ounces) chickpeas, rinsed and drained
- 1 ripe avocado, diced
- 1 small red onion, finely chopped
- 1 cucumber, diced
- 1 red bell pepper, diced
- 1/4 cup fresh cilantro, chopped
- 2 tablespoons olive oil
- Juice of 1 lime
- Salt and pepper, to taste

Instructions:

1. In a large bowl, combine the chickpeas, avocado, red onion, cucumber, and red bell pepper.

2. Add the chopped cilantro to the bowl.

3. In a small bowl, whisk together the olive oil and lime juice with a pinch of salt and pepper to create the dressing.

4. Pour the dressing over the salad ingredients and gently toss to combine. Make sure all ingredients are evenly coated.

5. Season the salad with additional salt and pepper according to taste.

6. Let the salad sit for about 10 minutes before serving to allow the flavors to meld.

Nutritional Information (per serving):

- Calories: 250
- Total Fat: 14g
- Saturated Fat: 2g
- Cholesterol: 0mg
- Sodium: 300mg
- Total Carbohydrates: 27g
- Dietary Fiber: 8g
- Sugars: 5g
- Protein: 7g

Serving Size: 1 cup

Cooking Time: 10 minutes (preparation time)

Chapter 4: Dinner Foods for Diabetics

Baked Cod with Roasted Vegetables

Ingredients:

- 4 cod fillets (6 ounces each)
- 2 tablespoons olive oil
- 1 teaspoon garlic powder
- 1 teaspoon dried basil
- 1/2 teaspoon salt
- 1/4 teaspoon black pepper
- 1 medium zucchini, sliced
- 1 red bell pepper, cut into 1-inch pieces
- 1 yellow bell pepper, cut into 1-inch pieces
- 1 small red onion, cut into wedges
- 1/2 cup cherry tomatoes
- 1 lemon, sliced for garnish
- Fresh parsley, chopped (for garnish)

Instructions:

1. Preheat the oven to 400°F (204°C). Line a large baking sheet with parchment paper.

2. Arrange the cod fillets in the center of the prepared baking sheet.

3. In a small bowl, mix olive oil, garlic powder, dried basil, salt, and black pepper. Brush half of this mixture over the cod fillets.

4. In a large bowl, combine the zucchini, red and yellow bell peppers, red onion, and cherry tomatoes. Toss the vegetables with the remaining olive oil mixture until well coated.

5. Spread the vegetables around the cod fillets on the baking sheet.

6. Bake in the preheated oven for 20-25 minutes, or until the cod flakes easily with a fork and the vegetables are tender.

7. Garnish with lemon slices and chopped fresh parsley before serving.

Nutritional Information:

- Calories: 240
- Total Fat: 10 g
- Saturated Fat: 1.5 g
- Cholesterol: 60 mg
- Sodium: 350 mg
- Total Carbohydrates: 10 g
- Dietary Fiber: 3 g
- Sugars: 5 g
- Protein: 28 g

Serving Size:

- This recipe serves 4 people.

Cooking Time:

- Preparation time: 10 minutes
- Cooking time: 25 minutes
- Total time: 35 minutes

Ingredients:

- 1 lb boneless, skinless chicken breast, thinly sliced
- 2 cups broccoli florets
- 1 red bell pepper, sliced into thin strips
- 1 carrot, thinly sliced
- 2 teaspoons olive oil
- 2 garlic cloves, minced
- 1 tablespoon ginger, freshly grated
- 1/4 cup low-sodium soy sauce
- 1 tablespoon sesame oil
- 1 teaspoon cornstarch
- 1/4 cup chicken broth (low sodium)
- Salt and pepper, to taste
- 1 tablespoon sesame seeds (optional, for garnish)

Instructions:

1. In a small bowl, whisk together the low-sodium soy sauce, sesame oil, cornstarch, and chicken broth. Set aside.
2. Heat the olive oil in a large skillet or wok over medium-high heat.
3. Add the garlic and ginger, sautéing for about 30 seconds until fragrant.
4. Increase the heat to high and add the chicken slices. Stir-fry for 3-4 minutes until the chicken is almost cooked through.

5. Add the broccoli, red bell pepper, and carrot to the skillet. Continue to stir-fry for an additional 5-7 minutes until the vegetables are tender and the chicken is fully cooked.

6. Reduce the heat to medium, pour the sauce mixture over the cooked chicken and vegetables, and stir well to combine. Cook for another 2-3 minutes until the sauce has thickened.

7. Season with salt and pepper to taste. Garnish with sesame seeds if desired.

Nutritional Information (per serving):

- Calories: 225
- Total Fat: 8g
- Saturated Fat: 1.5g
- Cholesterol: 65mg
- Sodium: 320mg
- Total Carbohydrates: 10g
- Dietary Fiber: 3g
- Sugars: 4g
- Protein: 29g

Serving Size: 4 servings

Cooking Time: 20 minutes

Eggplant Parmesan with Marinara
Sauce

Ingredients:

- 1 large eggplant, sliced into 1/2-inch thick rounds
- 2 cups marinara sauce, no sugar added
- 1 cup shredded mozzarella cheese, part-skim
- 1/2 cup grated Parmesan cheese
- 1/2 cup whole wheat breadcrumbs
- 2 large eggs, beaten
- 1/4 cup fresh basil leaves, chopped
- 2 cloves garlic, minced
- Olive oil for brushing
- Salt and pepper to taste

Instructions:

1. Preheat your oven to 375°F (190°C). Lightly grease a baking sheet with olive oil.

2. Season eggplant slices with salt and let them sit for about 20 minutes to draw out moisture. Pat dry with paper towels.

3. Dip eggplant slices in beaten eggs, then coat with breadcrumbs mixed with minced garlic and a pinch of pepper.

4. Place coated eggplant slices on the prepared baking sheet and lightly brush the tops with olive oil.

5. Bake in the preheated oven for 20 minutes, turning once until the eggplant is golden and crispy.

6. In a baking dish, spread a thin layer of marinara sauce. Arrange a layer of baked eggplant slices over the sauce. Sprinkle with mozzarella and Parmesan cheeses. Repeat the layers until all the eggplant slices are used.
7. Top the final layer with the remaining marinara sauce and cheeses.
8. Bake in the oven for 20-25 minutes, or until the cheese is bubbly and golden brown.
9. Garnish with fresh basil before serving.

Nutritional Information (per serving):

- Calories: 250
- Carbohydrates: 18g
- Fiber: 6g
- Protein: 15g
- Fat: 14g
- Sodium: 450mg

Serving Size: 1/4 of the dish

Cooking Time: 40-45 minutes (prep time: 15 minutes, cook time: 25-30 minutes)

Turkey Chili with Beans

Ingredients:

- 1 tablespoon olive oil
- 1 medium onion, diced
- 2 cloves garlic, minced
- 1 pound ground turkey
- 1 can (15 ounces) kidney beans, rinsed and drained
- 1 can (15 ounces) black beans, rinsed and drained
- 1 can (15 ounces) diced tomatoes, with juice
- 1 cup low-sodium chicken broth
- 1 tablespoon chili powder
- 1 teaspoon ground cumin
- 1 teaspoon paprika
- 1/2 teaspoon dried oregano
- 1/2 teaspoon salt
- 1/4 teaspoon ground black pepper
- 1/4 teaspoon cayenne pepper (optional, for extra heat)
- 1/2 cup chopped fresh cilantro (optional, for garnish)
- 1/2 cup shredded reduced-fat cheddar cheese (optional, for garnish)

Instructions:

1. In a large pot, heat olive oil over medium heat. Add the diced onion and cook until it becomes translucent, about 5 minutes.

Add minced garlic and cook for an additional 1-2 minutes until fragrant.

2. Add ground turkey to the pot and cook until browned, breaking it up with a spoon as it cooks, about 7-8 minutes.

3. Stir in kidney beans, black beans, diced tomatoes (with their juice), and chicken broth.

4. Add chili powder, ground cumin, paprika, dried oregano, salt, black pepper, and cayenne pepper (if using). Stir to combine.

5. Bring the mixture to a boil, then reduce heat to low and simmer, uncovered, for 30-35 minutes, stirring occasionally.

6. Taste and adjust seasonings as needed.

7. Serve hot, garnished with chopped cilantro and shredded cheddar cheese, if desired.

Nutritional Information (per serving):

- Calories: 250
- Total Fat: 8g
- Saturated Fat: 2g
- Cholesterol: 50mg
- Sodium: 450mg
- Total Carbohydrates: 24g
- Dietary Fiber: 8g
- Sugars: 4g
- Protein: 22g

Serving Size: 1 cup

Cooking Time: 45-50 minutes

Ingredients:

- 4 medium zucchinis, spiralized into noodles
- 1 cup fresh basil leaves
- 1/4 cup pine nuts
- 1/4 cup grated Parmesan cheese
- 2 cloves garlic, minced
- 1/4 cup extra-virgin olive oil
- Salt and pepper to taste
- 1 tablespoon lemon juice

Instructions:

1. Prepare the Pesto: In a food processor, combine basil leaves, pine nuts, Parmesan cheese, and garlic. Pulse until the mixture is finely chopped.

2. Add Olive Oil: With the processor running, slowly add the olive oil until the mixture is smooth. Add lemon juice, and season with salt and pepper to taste.

3. Cook Zucchini Noodles: In a large skillet, heat a small amount of olive oil over medium heat. Add the spiralized zucchini noodles and sauté for 3-4 minutes until just tender, but not mushy.

4. Combine: Remove the skillet from heat and toss the zucchini noodles with the prepared pesto until evenly coated.

5. Serve: Transfer to serving plates and garnish with additional pine nuts and grated Parmesan cheese if desired.

Nutritional Information (per serving):

- Calories: 220
- Total Fat: 19g
- Saturated Fat: 3g
- Cholesterol: 5mg
- Sodium: 120mg
- Total Carbohydrates: 7g
- Dietary Fiber: 2g
- Sugars: 5g
- Protein: 5g

Serving Size: 2 cups of zucchini noodles

Cooking Time: 15 minutes

Pork Tenderloin with Apple Cider Glaze

Ingredients:

- 1 ½ pounds pork tenderloin, trimmed
- 1 cup apple cider
- 1 tablespoon Dijon mustard
- 1 tablespoon apple cider vinegar
- 2 teaspoons olive oil
- 2 garlic cloves, minced
- 1 teaspoon dried thyme
- 1 teaspoon dried rosemary
- Salt and pepper to taste

Instructions:

1. **Prepare the Pork Tenderloin:**
   - Preheat your oven to 375°F (190°C).
   - Season the pork tenderloin with salt and pepper.
   - In a large ovenproof skillet, heat the olive oil over medium-high heat.
   - Sear the pork tenderloin on all sides until browned, about 3-4 minutes per side.

2. **Make the Glaze:**
   - In a small bowl, whisk together the apple cider, Dijon mustard, apple cider vinegar, garlic, thyme, and rosemary.

3. **Cook the Pork Tenderloin:**

   - Pour the apple cider mixture over the pork tenderloin in the skillet.

   - Transfer the skillet to the preheated oven.

   - Roast the pork tenderloin for about 20-25 minutes, or until the internal temperature reaches 145°F (63°C).

4. **Rest and Serve:**

   - Remove the skillet from the oven and transfer the pork tenderloin to a cutting board.

   - Let the pork rest for 5-10 minutes before slicing.

   - Slice the pork tenderloin and drizzle with the apple cider glaze from the skillet.

Nutritional Information (per serving):

- Calories: 220
- Protein: 26g
- Carbohydrates: 5g
- Dietary Fiber: 0g
- Sugars: 3g
- Total Fat: 10g
- Saturated Fat: 2g
- Cholesterol: 75mg
- Sodium: 300mg

Serving Size:

- Serves 4

Cooking Time:

- Total: 35-40 minutes

Ingredients:

- 1 block firm tofu, drained and pressed
- 2 large sweet potatoes, peeled and diced
- 1 bunch kale, stems removed and leaves chopped
- 2 tablespoons olive oil
- 1 teaspoon garlic powder
- 1 teaspoon onion powder
- 1 teaspoon smoked paprika
- 1 teaspoon dried thyme
- 1 tablespoon soy sauce (low-sodium)
- 1 tablespoon balsamic vinegar
- Salt and pepper to taste

Instructions:

1. Preheat your oven to 400°F (200°C).
2. Cut the pressed tofu into 1-inch cubes and place them in a bowl.
3. In a small bowl, mix together the olive oil, garlic powder, onion powder, smoked paprika, dried thyme, soy sauce, and balsamic vinegar.
4. Pour half of the marinade over the tofu cubes, tossing gently to coat. Let it marinate for at least 15 minutes.

5. In another bowl, toss the sweet potatoes with the remaining marinade.

6. Spread the sweet potatoes evenly on a baking sheet lined with parchment paper. Bake in the preheated oven for 20 minutes.

7. After 20 minutes, add the marinated tofu to the baking sheet with the sweet potatoes. Bake for an additional 15-20 minutes or until the tofu is golden and the sweet potatoes are tender.

8. While the tofu and sweet potatoes are baking, heat a large skillet over medium heat. Add the chopped kale and a splash of water. Cook, stirring occasionally, until the kale is wilted and tender, about 5 minutes. Season with salt and pepper to taste.

9. Serve the baked tofu and sweet potatoes over a bed of wilted kale.

Nutritional Information (per serving):

- Calories: 250
- Protein: 12g
- Carbohydrates: 30g
- Dietary Fiber: 6g
- Sugars: 8g
- Fat: 10g
- Saturated Fat: 1.5g
- Sodium: 320mg
- Potassium: 750mg

Serving Size:

- Serves 4

Cooking Time:

- Total: 45-50 minutes
  - Prep Time: 15 minutes
  - Cook Time: 30-35 minutes

Ingredients:

- 1 lb lean beef stew meat, cut into 1-inch cubes
- 2 tbsp olive oil
- 1 large onion, chopped
- 2 garlic cloves, minced
- 4 cups low-sodium beef broth
- 2 large carrots, peeled and cut into chunks
- 2 large parsnips, peeled and cut into chunks
- 2 medium turnips, peeled and cut into chunks
- 1 large sweet potato, peeled and cut into chunks
- 1 tsp dried thyme
- 1 tsp dried rosemary
- 2 bay leaves
- Salt and pepper to taste
- 1/4 cup fresh parsley, chopped (for garnish)

Instructions:

1. **Prepare the Beef:** In a large pot or Dutch oven, heat the olive oil over medium-high heat. Add the beef cubes in batches, making sure not to overcrowd the pot. Brown the beef on all sides, about 5-7 minutes per batch. Remove the beef from the pot and set aside.

2. **Sauté Aromatics:** In the same pot, add the chopped onion and sauté until it becomes translucent, about 5 minutes. Add the minced garlic and cook for an additional 1-2 minutes, stirring frequently to prevent burning.

3. **Combine Ingredients:** Return the browned beef to the pot. Pour in the beef broth, making sure to scrape the bottom of the pot to release any browned bits (these add flavor). Add the carrots, parsnips, turnips, sweet potato, thyme, rosemary, and bay leaves. Stir to combine.

4. **Simmer:** Bring the mixture to a boil, then reduce the heat to low. Cover the pot and let the stew simmer for 1.5 to 2 hours, or until the beef and vegetables are tender. Stir occasionally to ensure even cooking.

5. **Season and Serve:** Remove the bay leaves from the stew. Taste and adjust seasoning with salt and pepper as needed. Ladle the stew into bowls and garnish with chopped fresh parsley.

Nutritional Information (per serving):

- Calories: 350
- Protein: 25g
- Carbohydrates: 25g
- Dietary Fiber: 5g
- Sugars: 7g

- Fat: 15g
- Saturated Fat: 4g
- Cholesterol: 75mg
- Sodium: 500mg

Serving Size:

- Makes 4 servings

Cooking Time:

- Preparation Time: 20 minutes
- Cooking Time: 1.5 to 2 hours

Ingredients:

- 4 large bell peppers (any color), tops cut off and seeds removed
- 1 cup quinoa, rinsed
- 2 cups low-sodium vegetable broth
- 1 tablespoon olive oil
- 1 medium onion, finely chopped
- 2 cloves garlic, minced
- 1 cup cherry tomatoes, halved
- 1 cup black beans, rinsed and drained
- 1 cup corn kernels (fresh, frozen, or canned)
- 1 teaspoon ground cumin
- 1 teaspoon smoked paprika
- 1/2 teaspoon ground black pepper
- 1/4 teaspoon salt
- 1/4 cup fresh cilantro, chopped
- 1 cup shredded reduced-fat mozzarella cheese

Instructions:

1. Preheat the oven to 375°F (190°C).
2. Cook the quinoa in the vegetable broth according to package instructions. Set aside.
3. In a large skillet, heat the olive oil over medium heat. Add the onion and garlic, sautéing until the onion is translucent, about 5 minutes.

4. Stir in the cherry tomatoes, black beans, corn, cumin, smoked paprika, black pepper, and salt. Cook for another 5 minutes, allowing the flavors to meld together.

5. Add the cooked quinoa to the skillet and mix well. Remove from heat and stir in the fresh cilantro.

6. Fill each bell pepper with the quinoa mixture, pressing down lightly to pack it in.

7. Place the stuffed peppers in a baking dish. Cover with foil and bake for 30 minutes.

8. Remove the foil, sprinkle the tops of the peppers with the shredded mozzarella cheese, and bake for an additional 10-15 minutes, until the cheese is melted and bubbly.

9. Let the stuffed peppers cool for a few minutes before serving.

Nutritional Information (per serving):

- Calories: 250
- Total Fat: 8g
- Saturated Fat: 2g
- Cholesterol: 10mg
- Sodium: 250mg
- Total Carbohydrates: 35g
- Dietary Fiber: 7g
- Sugars: 6g
- Protein: 10g

Serving Size: 1 stuffed bell pepper

Cooking Time: 50-55 minutes

Ingredients:

- 1 cup fresh spinach, finely chopped
- 1 cup ricotta cheese (part-skim)
- 1/4 cup grated Parmesan cheese
- 1 large egg
- 1/2 teaspoon salt
- 1/4 teaspoon black pepper
- 1/4 teaspoon nutmeg
- 1 package of whole wheat ravioli dough or wonton wrappers
- 2 tablespoons olive oil
- 2 cloves garlic, minced
- 1 cup low-sodium tomato sauce
- Fresh basil leaves for garnish

Instructions:

1. **Prepare the Filling:**

   - In a mixing bowl, combine the chopped spinach, ricotta cheese, Parmesan cheese, egg, salt, pepper, and nutmeg. Mix well until all ingredients are evenly distributed.

2. **Assemble the Ravioli:**

   - If using whole wheat ravioli dough, roll it out on a lightly floured surface to about 1/8 inch thickness. If using wonton wrappers, lay them out on a clean surface.

- Place a teaspoon of the spinach and ricotta mixture in the center of each dough piece or wonton wrapper.

- Lightly brush the edges with water, then fold the dough over to create a half-moon shape (or seal with another wrapper if using wonton wrappers), pressing the edges firmly to seal. Ensure there are no air pockets.

3. **Cook the Ravioli:**

- Bring a large pot of salted water to a gentle boil. Carefully add the ravioli in batches, cooking for about 3-4 minutes or until they float to the top.

- Remove with a slotted spoon and set aside.

4. **Prepare the Sauce:**

- In a large skillet, heat the olive oil over medium heat. Add the minced garlic and sauté until fragrant, about 1 minute.

- Add the low-sodium tomato sauce to the skillet and simmer for 5-7 minutes, stirring occasionally.

5. **Combine and Serve:**

- Gently add the cooked ravioli to the skillet with the tomato sauce, stirring carefully to coat the ravioli evenly.

- Garnish with fresh basil leaves before serving.

Nutritional Information (per serving):

- Calories: 320

- Total Fat: 15g

- Saturated Fat: 5g

- Cholesterol: 60mg

- Sodium: 420mg

- Total Carbohydrates: 30g

- Dietary Fiber: 4g

- Sugars: 4g

- Protein: 15g

Serving Size:

- Serves 4

Cooking Time:

- Total: 30 minutes
  - Preparation: 15 minutes
  - Cooking: 15 minutes

Chapter 5: Snacks and Desserts

Ingredients:

- 1 cup plain Greek yogurt

- 1/2 cup fresh berries (strawberries, blueberries, or raspberries)

- 1 tablespoon chia seeds

- 1 teaspoon honey (optional)

Instructions:

1. In a bowl, combine the Greek yogurt and fresh berries.

2. Sprinkle chia seeds on top.

3. Drizzle honey over the mixture if desired.

4. Mix well and serve immediately.

Nutritional Information (per serving):

- Calories: 180

- Carbohydrates: 15g

- Protein: 15g

- Fat: 6g

- Fiber: 5g

Serving Size: 1 bowl

Cooking Time: 5 minutes

Apple Slices with Peanut Butter

Ingredients:

- 1 medium apple, sliced
- 2 tablespoons natural peanut butter

Instructions:

1. Wash and slice the apple into thin wedges.
2. Spread peanut butter evenly over each apple slice.
3. Serve immediately.

Nutritional Information (per serving):

- Calories: 190
- Carbohydrates: 22g
- Protein: 4g
- Fat: 9g
- Fiber: 4g

Serving Size: 1 apple with peanut butter

Cooking Time: 5 minutes

Hummus and Veggie Sticks

Ingredients:

- 1/2 cup hummus

- 1 carrot, cut into sticks

- 1 celery stalk, cut into sticks

- 1 cucumber, sliced

Instructions:

1. Arrange the carrot, celery, and cucumber sticks on a plate.

2. Place the hummus in a small bowl.

3. Dip the veggie sticks into the hummus and enjoy.

Nutritional Information (per serving):

- Calories: 150

- Carbohydrates: 17g

- Protein: 5g

- Fat: 8g

- Fiber: 5g

Serving Size: 1 plate of veggies with hummus

Cooking Time: 10 minutes

Chia Pudding

Ingredients:

- 1/4 cup chia seeds

- 1 cup unsweetened almond milk
- 1 teaspoon vanilla extract
- 1 tablespoon honey (optional)
- Fresh berries for topping

Instructions:

1. In a bowl, mix chia seeds, almond milk, vanilla extract, and honey.
2. Stir well and refrigerate for at least 2 hours, or overnight.
3. Top with fresh berries before serving.

Nutritional Information (per serving):
- Calories: 200
- Carbohydrates: 24g
- Protein: 6g
- Fat: 8g
- Fiber: 10g

Serving Size: 1 cup

Cooking Time: 5 minutes (plus refrigeration time)

Dark Chocolate Almonds

Ingredients:
- 1/2 cup raw almonds

- 2 ounces dark chocolate (70% cocoa or higher), melted

Instructions:

1. Line a baking sheet with parchment paper.

2. Dip each almond into the melted dark chocolate.

3. Place the chocolate-covered almonds on the parchment paper.

4. Refrigerate until the chocolate hardens, about 15 minutes.

5. Serve immediately or store in an airtight container.

Nutritional Information (per serving):

- Calories: 250
- Carbohydrates: 15g
- Protein: 6g
- Fat: 20g
- Fiber: 5g

Serving Size: 1/4 cup

Cooking Time: 20 minutes

Cottage Cheese with Pineapple

Ingredients:

- 1 cup low-fat cottage cheese
- 1/2 cup pineapple chunks (fresh or canned in juice, drained)

Instructions:

1. In a bowl, combine the cottage cheese and pineapple chunks.

2. Mix well and serve immediately.

Nutritional Information (per serving):

- Calories: 160

- Carbohydrates: 18g

- Protein: 14g

- Fat: 2g

- Fiber: 2g

Serving Size: 1 bowl

Cooking Time: 5 minutes

Frozen Yogurt Bark

Ingredients:

- 2 cups plain Greek yogurt

- 1/2 cup fresh berries (blueberries, raspberries, or strawberries)

- 1/4 cup chopped nuts (almonds or walnuts)

- 1 tablespoon honey (optional)

Instructions:

1. Line a baking sheet with parchment paper.

2. Spread the Greek yogurt evenly over the parchment paper.

3. Sprinkle the berries and chopped nuts on top.

4. Drizzle honey over the mixture if desired.

5. Freeze for at least 2 hours, or until firm.

6. Break into pieces and serve.

Nutritional Information (per serving):

- Calories: 120

- Carbohydrates: 12g

- Protein: 10g

- Fat: 5g

- Fiber: 3g

Serving Size: 1/4 of the bark

Cooking Time: 2 hours (freezing time)

Apple Slices with Almond Butter

Ingredients:

- 1 medium apple, sliced
- 2 tablespoons almond butter

Instructions:

1. Wash and slice the apple into thin wedges.
2. Spread almond butter on each apple slice.
3. Serve immediately.

Nutritional Information (Per Serving):

- Calories: 180
- Carbohydrates: 22g
- Fiber: 5g
- Protein: 4g
- Fat: 10g

Serving Size: 1 apple with 2 tablespoons almond butter

Cooking Time: 5 minutes

Greek Yogurt with Berries

Ingredients:

- 1 cup plain Greek yogurt
- 1/2 cup mixed berries (strawberries, blueberries, raspberries)
- 1 teaspoon honey (optional)

Instructions:

1. Spoon the Greek yogurt into a bowl.
2. Top with mixed berries.
3. Drizzle honey over the top if desired.
4. Serve chilled.

Nutritional Information (Per Serving):

- Calories: 150
- Carbohydrates: 18g
- Fiber: 3g
- Protein: 12g
  Fat: 4g

Serving Size: 1 cup yogurt with 1/2 cup berries

Cooking Time: 5 minutes

Chia Seed Pudding

Ingredients:

- 1/4 cup chia seeds
- 1 cup unsweetened almond milk
- 1 teaspoon vanilla extract
- 1 tablespoon maple syrup (optional)
- Fresh berries for topping

Instructions:

1. In a bowl, combine chia seeds, almond milk, vanilla extract, and maple syrup.
2. Stir well until chia seeds are evenly distributed.
3. Refrigerate for at least 4 hours or overnight.
4. Stir the pudding and top with fresh berries before serving.

Nutritional Information (Per Serving):
- Calories: 200
- Carbohydrates: 20g
- Fiber: 10g
- Protein: 5g
- Fat: 10g

Serving Size: 1 cup chia seed pudding

Cooking Time: 10 minutes prep, 4 hours refrigeration

Dark Chocolate Almond Bark

Ingredients:

- 1 cup dark chocolate chips (70% cacao or higher)
- 1/2 cup almonds, chopped
- 1 teaspoon sea salt

Instructions:

1. Melt the dark chocolate chips in a microwave-safe bowl in 30-second intervals, stirring each time, until fully melted.
2. Stir in the chopped almonds.
3. Spread the mixture onto a parchment-lined baking sheet into an even layer.
4. Sprinkle sea salt over the top.
5. Refrigerate until set, about 30 minutes.
6. Break into pieces and serve.

Nutritional Information (Per Serving):

- Calories: 150
- Carbohydrates: 12g
- Fiber: 3g
- Protein: 3g
- Fat: 10g

Serving Size: 1 ounce of bark

Cooking Time: 10 minutes prep, 30 minutes refrigeration

Conclusion

Managing diabetes effectively, especially after the age of 50, requires a well-balanced and thoughtful approach to nutrition. "The Complete Diabetic Diet After 50" provides a comprehensive guide to making informed dietary choices that promote stable blood sugar levels, overall health, and well-being. Here are the key takeaways from this guide:

Emphasis on Balanced Meals

A central theme of this guide is the importance of balanced meals. Incorporating a variety of nutrient-dense foods ensures that you receive essential vitamins and minerals while maintaining blood sugar control. Meals should include:

- **Lean Proteins:** Such as poultry, fish, tofu, and legumes.
- Healthy Fats: Found in avocados, nuts, seeds, and olive oil.
- **Fiber-Rich Carbohydrates:** Including whole grains, fruits, and vegetables.
- **Low Glycemic Index Foods:** To prevent rapid spikes in blood sugar.

Importance of Regular Monitoring

Consistent monitoring of blood sugar levels helps in understanding how different foods affect your body. This guide underscores the significance of:

- **Frequent Blood Glucose Testing:** To identify patterns and make necessary dietary adjustments.
- Professional Consultations: Regular check-ins with healthcare providers to optimize your diabetes management plan.

Smart Snacking and Desserts

Healthy snacking and dessert options are not only permissible but encouraged. By choosing nutrient-dense snacks and desserts that are low in sugar and high in fiber and healthy fats, you can enjoy treats without compromising your blood sugar control. Key strategies include:

- **Portion Control**: Keeping snacks and desserts in moderation.
- **Ingredient Choices:** Opting for natural sweeteners, whole grains, and healthy fats.

Meal Planning and Preparation

Effective meal planning is crucial for managing diabetes. Planning meals ahead of time helps ensure that you always have healthy options available, reducing the temptation to opt for less healthy, convenience foods. Tips include:

- **Batch Cooking:** Preparing meals in advance to save time and ensure consistency.
- **Diverse Menus:** Keeping meals varied to prevent dietary boredom and ensure a range of nutrients.

Lifestyle Integration

Diet is a fundamental aspect of diabetes management, but it is also important to integrate other healthy lifestyle habits:

- **Regular Physical Activity:** Engaging in at least 150 minutes of moderate exercise per week.
- **Hydration:** Drinking plenty of water throughout the day.
- Adequate Sleep: Ensuring you get 7-9 hours of sleep per night.

Final Thoughts

"The Complete Diabetic Diet After 50" aims to empower you with the knowledge and tools needed to take control of your health through mindful eating and lifestyle choices. By focusing on balanced nutrition, regular monitoring, smart snacking, and integrating healthy habits into your daily routine, you can effectively manage your diabetes and enhance your quality of life.

Remember, each small step you take towards healthier eating and living contributes significantly to your overall well-being.